Contents

Chapter 1: Introduction to Chair Yoga for Seniors

As we age, our bodies change, and we may begin to experience physical limitations that can make it more difficult to maintain an active lifestyle. Yoga is an excellent way to stay active and healthy, but many seniors may find traditional yoga classes too challenging. That's where chair yoga comes in.

Chair yoga is a gentle form of yoga that is accessible to people of all ages and abilities. It is a seated practice that uses a chair for support, making it ideal for seniors who may have balance issues, mobility limitations, or difficulty getting up and down from the floor.

The benefits of chair yoga are many. It can improve flexibility, strength, balance, and mobility, while also reducing stress and anxiety. It is a low-impact exercise that is gentle on the joints, making it an excellent choice for seniors who may have arthritis or other joint-related issues.

In this chapter, we'll take a closer look at what chair yoga is, how it differs from traditional yoga, and why it's such a great option for seniors.

What is Chair Yoga?

Chair yoga is a modified form of yoga that is done while sitting on a chair or using a chair for support. It incorporates traditional yoga poses, breathing exercises, and meditation, but is adapted to make it accessible to people who may have difficulty with traditional yoga practices.

In chair yoga, the chair becomes an extension of your body, allowing you to perform poses that might be difficult or impossible to do on your own. The chair provides support, stability, and balance, allowing you to move safely and comfortably through the poses.

Chair yoga is highly adaptable and can be modified to suit the needs and abilities of each individual practitioner. The poses can be done slowly and gently, or more vigorously if desired. The focus is on finding a comfortable and safe range of motion, rather than pushing yourself to your limits.

How is Chair Yoga Different from Traditional Yoga?

While chair yoga incorporates many of the same principles as traditional yoga, there are some key differences that make it more accessible for seniors. Here are a few ways that chair yoga differs from traditional yoga:

- Chair yoga is done while sitting on a chair or using a chair for support. Traditional yoga is typically done on a yoga mat on the floor.

- Chair yoga poses are modified to make them accessible to seniors with mobility limitations or other physical challenges.

Traditional yoga poses may be more advanced and require more strength and flexibility.

- In chair yoga, the focus is on finding a comfortable and safe range of motion, rather than pushing yourself to your limits. Traditional yoga may be more challenging and require more effort and stamina.

- Chair yoga incorporates breathing exercises and meditation but may place more emphasis on these practices than traditional yoga.

Why is Chair Yoga a Great Option for Seniors?

There are many reasons why chair yoga is an excellent option for seniors. Here are a few of the key benefits:

- Chair yoga is gentle and low-impact, making it safe for seniors who may have arthritis, osteoporosis, or other joint-related issues.

- Chair yoga can improve flexibility, strength, balance, and mobility, which are all important for maintaining independence and reducing the risk of falls.

- Chair yoga is adaptable to individual needs and abilities, making it a great option for seniors who may have physical limitations or chronic conditions.

- Chair yoga can reduce stress and anxiety, improve mood, and promote a sense of well-being.

- Chair yoga can be done anywhere, making it convenient and accessible for seniors who may not be able to attend traditional yoga classes.

Chair yoga is a gentle and accessible form of yoga that is ideal for seniors. It offers many benefits, including improved flexibility, strength, balance, and mobility, as well as reduced stress and anxiety. It is highly adaptable, making it a great option for seniors who may have physical limitations or chronic conditions.

In the next chapter, we'll explore the specific benefits of chair yoga for seniors in more detail, including how it can improve joint health, balance, and overall well-being. We'll also provide tips for getting started with chair yoga, including how to find a qualified instructor, what to look for in a chair, and how to create a safe and comfortable practice space.

Whether you're a senior looking to maintain your health and independence, or a caregiver or healthcare provider looking for ways to support the well-being of your elderly clients or loved ones, chair yoga is an excellent option to consider. With its gentle, adaptable approach and numerous benefits, it is a practice that can help seniors stay healthy and active for years to come.

Chapter 2: Benefits of Chair Yoga for Seniors

Chair yoga is a gentle and accessible form of yoga that provides many benefits for seniors. In this chapter, we'll explore some of the specific ways that chair yoga can improve the health and well-being of older adults.

Improves Joint Health

One of the primary benefits of chair yoga for seniors is improved joint health. As we age, our joints can become stiff and less flexible, which can lead to pain, discomfort, and reduced mobility. Chair yoga can help to alleviate these symptoms by improving joint mobility and flexibility.

Chair yoga poses gently stretch and strengthen the muscles around the joints, increasing their range of motion and reducing stiffness. This can be especially beneficial for seniors with arthritis, who may experience pain and inflammation in their joints. Chair yoga can also help to reduce the risk of falls by improving balance and coordination.

Promotes Cardiovascular Health

Cardiovascular disease is a leading cause of death among seniors. Regular exercise can help to reduce the risk of cardiovascular disease by improving heart health and circulation. Chair yoga can provide a gentle form of cardiovascular exercise for seniors who may not be able to engage in more vigorous activities.

Many chair yoga poses involve deep breathing and rhythmic movement, which can improve circulation and increase oxygenation of the blood. This can help to lower blood pressure and reduce the risk of heart disease.

Reduces Stress and Anxiety

Stress and anxiety can have a negative impact on overall health and well-being, especially for seniors who may be dealing with chronic health conditions or other age-related challenges. Chair yoga can help to reduce stress and anxiety by promoting relaxation and mindfulness.

Chair yoga incorporates breathing techniques and meditation practices that can help to calm the mind and reduce feelings of stress and anxiety. By focusing on the present moment and letting go of worries and concerns, seniors can experience greater peace and tranquility in their daily lives.

Improves Mood and Mental Health

In addition to reducing stress and anxiety, chair yoga can also improve mood and overall mental health. Regular practice of chair yoga has been shown to improve symptoms of depression and increase feelings of happiness and well-being.

Chair yoga can also provide a sense of community and social connection for seniors, who may be dealing with feelings of isolation or loneliness. Group chair yoga classes can be a great way to meet new people and connect with others who share similar interests and challenges.

Increases Strength and Balance

Maintaining strength and balance is crucial for seniors to prevent falls and maintain independence. Chair yoga can help to improve strength and balance by gently strengthening the muscles and improving coordination.

Many chair yoga poses involve holding and supporting the body's weight, which can help to build strength in the muscles of the arms, legs, and core. Chair yoga can also improve balance by focusing on the alignment and stability of the body in each pose.

Chair yoga provides many benefits for seniors, including improved joint health, cardiovascular health, stress reduction, improved mood, and increased strength and balance. By incorporating chair yoga into their daily routine, seniors can experience greater health and well-being, and maintain their independence and vitality for years to come. In the next chapter, we'll provide tips for getting started with chair yoga, including finding a qualified instructor and creating a safe and comfortable practice space.

Chapter 3: Understanding the Basics of Yoga

Before delving into the specific practices of chair yoga, it's important to have a basic understanding of yoga as a whole. Yoga is an ancient practice that originated in India thousands of years ago. It is a holistic approach to health and well-being that involves physical postures, breathing techniques, meditation, and ethical principles.

Physical Postures (Asanas)

The physical postures, or asanas, are what most people think of when they hear the word "yoga". These are the poses that are practiced in a yoga class, and they can range from simple, seated poses to complex, challenging postures that require strength and flexibility.

The practice of asanas is designed to improve physical health and well-being by stretching and strengthening the muscles, increasing flexibility, and improving joint health. The physical postures also help to calm the mind and reduce stress by promoting mindfulness and focus.

Breathing Techniques (Pranayama)

Breathing techniques, or pranayama, are an essential part of yoga practice. The breath is seen as a vital force that connects the body and mind, and by controlling the breath, practitioners can control their mental and emotional state.

Pranayama techniques involve conscious manipulation of the breath, such as deep breathing, breath retention, and alternate nostril breathing. These techniques can help to calm the mind, reduce stress, and improve overall health and well-being.

Meditation (Dhyana)

Meditation is a key aspect of yoga practice that involves focusing the mind and cultivating inner awareness. Through meditation, practitioners can develop greater clarity, concentration, and insight into their own thoughts and emotions.

Meditation techniques can range from simple breathing exercises to more complex visualizations and mindfulness practices. The goal of meditation is to quiet the mind and cultivate a sense of inner peace and tranquility.

Ethical Principles (Yamas and Niyamas)

Yoga also includes a set of ethical principles, known as the yamas and niyamas, that provide guidance for living a virtuous and fulfilling life. These principles include concepts such as non-violence, honesty, and self-discipline.

By practicing these principles, yoga practitioners can cultivate greater self-awareness and compassion for themselves and others. The ethical principles of yoga are meant to be applied both on and off the mat and can help to promote greater harmony and peace in the world.

Yoga is a holistic practice that encompasses physical, mental, and spiritual aspects of health and well-being. By understanding the basic principles of yoga, including the physical postures, breathing techniques, meditation, and ethical principles, seniors can gain a deeper appreciation for the benefits of chair yoga practice.

In the next chapter, we'll provide tips for getting started with chair yoga, including finding a qualified instructor and creating a safe and comfortable practice space.

Chapter 4: Getting Started with Chair Yoga

Now that you have a basic understanding of yoga, it's time to start exploring chair yoga specifically. Chair yoga is a modified form of yoga that is practiced while seated in a chair, making it accessible for seniors or anyone with limited mobility or balance issues.

If you're new to yoga, it's important to start slowly and listen to your body. Here are some tips for getting started with chair yoga:

1. Find a Qualified Instructor

To ensure that you're practicing safely and effectively, it's important to find a qualified chair yoga instructor. Look for someone who has experience working with seniors or individuals with limited mobility, and who is knowledgeable about modifications and adjustments for different levels of ability.

You can find chair yoga classes at local community centres, senior centres, or yoga studios. If you prefer to practice at home, there are also many online chair yoga classes and tutorials available.

2. Create a Comfortable Practice Space

When practicing chair yoga, it's important to create a safe and comfortable practice space. Choose a sturdy chair without wheels, and make sure it is placed on a stable surface. You may also want to place a non-slip mat or blanket on the floor beneath the chair to provide extra stability.

Wear comfortable, loose-fitting clothing that allows for ease of movement. You may also want to have a small pillow or cushion available for added support.

3. Start with Simple Poses

Begin your practice with simple poses that focus on gentle stretching and breathing. Chair yoga poses can range from seated forward folds to seated twists and side stretches.

As you become more comfortable with the poses, you can gradually increase the intensity and duration of your practice. Always listen to your body and avoid any poses that cause pain or discomfort.

4. Practice Mindful Breathing

Breathing is a key aspect of chair yoga practice. Focus on slow, deep breathing, inhaling through your nose and exhaling through your mouth. You can also incorporate simple pranayama techniques, such as counting your breath or practicing alternate nostril breathing.

By practicing mindful breathing, you can calm the mind and reduce stress and anxiety.

5. Set Realistic Goals

As with any form of exercise, it's important to set realistic goals for your chair yoga practice. Start with a few minutes of practice each day and gradually increase the duration and intensity of your practice.

Remember that the benefits of chair yoga practice are cumulative, and even a few minutes of practice each day can lead to improved physical and mental well-being over time.

Chair yoga is a gentle and accessible form of yoga that can be practiced by seniors or anyone with limited mobility or balance issues. By finding a qualified instructor, creating a comfortable practice space, starting with simple poses, practicing mindful breathing, and setting realistic goals, you can enjoy the benefits of chair yoga practice at any age or ability level.

Chapter 5: Finding the Right Chair and Props

One of the great things about chair yoga is that it can be done almost anywhere, using any chair. However, there are some factors to consider when selecting the right chair and props to support your practice.

Choosing the Right Chair

When selecting a chair for chair yoga practice, it's important to choose one that is sturdy, comfortable, and the right size for your body. Here are some tips for finding the right chair:

1. Look for a Stable Chair

Choose a chair that is sturdy and doesn't wobble or tip over easily. The chair should be able to support your weight and provide a stable base for your practice.

2. Consider the Chair Height

The height of the chair is also important. Choose a chair that allows your feet to rest flat on the ground when seated. If the chair is too high, you may strain your legs and feet, and if it's too low, you may have difficulty getting up and down.

3. Choose a Comfortable Seat

Choose a chair with a comfortable seat that provides enough cushioning and support for your body. A chair with a padded seat or backrest can help to prevent discomfort or pain during your practice.

4. Avoid Chairs with Wheels

Avoid using chairs with wheels for chair yoga practice, as they can move or tip over easily and are not stable enough for certain poses.

5. Consider a Folding Chair

A folding chair can be a good option for chair yoga practice, as it can be easily transported and stored when not in use.

Props for Chair Yoga Practice

In addition to a sturdy chair, there are several props that can be used to support your chair yoga practice. Here are some common props and their uses:

1. Blankets

Blankets can be used to cushion the seat or back of the chair for added comfort, or as support for the knees or feet during certain poses.

2. Blocks

Blocks can be used to support the hands or feet during certain poses, or to bring the ground closer to the body for those with limited mobility.

3. Straps

Straps can be used to extend the reach of the arms during certain poses, or to support the legs or feet during seated forward folds.

4. Bolsters

Bolsters can be used to support the back, neck, or knees during restorative or gentle poses, and can provide added comfort and relaxation.

Choosing the right chair and props for your chair yoga practice can help to ensure safety, comfort, and support during your practice. When selecting a chair, look for a sturdy, comfortable, and appropriately sized chair that can provide a stable base for your practice. Use props such as blankets, blocks, straps, and bolsters to enhance your practice and support your body during poses. With the right equipment and props, you can enjoy the benefits of chair yoga practice with ease and comfort.

Chapter 6: Creating a Safe Environment for Chair Yoga

Creating a safe environment is essential for any yoga practice, and chair yoga is no exception. When practicing chair yoga, there are several factors to consider ensuring the safety and well-being of yourself and your students. In this chapter, we'll explore some key elements for creating a safe environment for chair yoga practice.

1. Clear Space

The first step in creating a safe environment for chair yoga practice is to clear the space of any potential hazards. Make sure that the area is free from clutter and that there is enough space to move around without bumping into any objects. If practicing in a group, make sure that each person has enough space to comfortably move their arms and legs without interfering with their neighbour.

2. Proper Lighting

Proper lighting is also important for chair yoga practice. Ensure that the space is well-lit, either with natural light or artificial lighting, to ensure that everyone can see what they are doing and avoid any potential tripping hazards.

3. Non-Slip Surface

It's important to practice on a non-slip surface to prevent slipping and falling during your practice. If practicing on a hard floor, consider placing a non-slip mat or rug under your chair to prevent it from moving or sliding during your practice.

4. Chairs and Props

As discussed in Chapter 5, choosing the right chair and props is important for safe and comfortable practice. Make sure that chairs are sturdy and the appropriate size for each participant. Provide enough props such as blankets, blocks, and straps to support participants in poses and ensure their safety.

5. Clear Instruction

Clear and concise instruction is crucial for safe and effective chair yoga practice. Provide step-by-step instructions for each pose, including modifications and variations, so that participants can adjust their practice to their individual needs and abilities. Encourage participants to listen to their bodies and avoid pushing themselves beyond their limits.

6. Breath Awareness

Breath awareness is an important aspect of any yoga practice, including chair yoga. Encourage participants to focus on their breath throughout their practice and to avoid holding their breath during poses. Deep breathing can help to calm the mind and relax the body and can also prevent dizziness and light-headedness during practice.

7. Physical Limitations

Be aware of any physical limitations or injuries that participants may have and provide modifications for poses as needed. Encourage participants to listen to their bodies and modify their practice accordingly to prevent injury and discomfort.

Creating a safe environment for chair yoga practice is essential for the well-being of yourself and your participants. Ensure that the space is clear and well-lit, use a non-slip surface, provide sturdy and appropriately sized chairs and props, and provide clear instruction and modifications for poses. Encourage participants to focus on their breath and listen to their bodies and be aware of any physical limitations or injuries. By creating a safe environment, participants can enjoy the benefits of chair yoga practice with ease and comfort.

Chapter 7: Breath Awareness and Control

Breath awareness and control are integral components of yoga practice, including chair yoga. In this chapter, we'll explore the importance of breath awareness and control in chair yoga and learn techniques for incorporating breath work into your practice.

The Importance of Breath Awareness and Control in Chair Yoga

Breath awareness and control are important for several reasons in chair yoga practice. First, breath awareness can help to calm the mind and reduce stress and anxiety. By focusing on the breath, we can bring our attention to the present moment and quiet the mind. This can help to improve mental clarity and reduce feelings of stress and overwhelm.

In addition to the mental benefits, breath control can also have physical benefits. By controlling our breath, we can increase oxygen intake, which can help to energize the body and improve circulation. Deep breathing can also help to activate the parasympathetic nervous system, which is responsible for promoting relaxation and reducing stress.

Breath awareness and control can also help to improve posture and spinal alignment in chair yoga practice. By focusing on the breath and maintaining steady, even breathing, we can increase our awareness of the alignment of our spine and ensure that we are sitting up straight and engaging our core muscles.

Breath Awareness Techniques in Chair Yoga

There are several techniques that can be used to increase breath awareness in chair yoga practice. Here are a few techniques to get started:

1. Diaphragmatic Breathing

Diaphragmatic breathing, also known as belly breathing, is a technique that involves breathing deeply into the belly rather than the chest. To practice diaphragmatic breathing, sit comfortably in your chair with your feet flat on the ground and your hands resting on your belly. Inhale deeply through your nose, filling your belly with air and feeling it expand. Exhale slowly through your mouth, feeling your belly deflate. Repeat for several breaths, focusing on the sensation of the breath moving in and out of your body.

2. Ujjayi Breathing

Ujjayi breathing is a technique that involves breathing in and out through the nose while constricting the muscles in the back of the throat. This produces a soft, audible sound similar to the sound of ocean waves. To practice ujjayi breathing, sit comfortably in your chair with your feet flat on the ground and your hands resting on your thighs. Inhale deeply through your nose while constricting the muscles in the back of your throat. Exhale slowly through your nose while maintaining the constriction in the throat. Repeat for several breaths, focusing on the sound of the breath and the sensation of the air moving in and out of your body.

3. Alternate Nostril Breathing

Alternate nostril breathing is a technique that involves breathing in and out through alternate nostrils. This technique is thought to balance the left and right hemispheres of the brain and promote relaxation. To practice alternate nostril breathing, sit comfortably in your chair with your feet flat on the ground and your hands resting on your thighs. Use your right thumb to close your right nostril and inhale deeply through your left nostril. Use your ring finger to close your left nostril and exhale slowly through your right nostril. Inhale deeply through your right nostril, then close your right nostril with your thumb and exhale slowly through your left nostril. Repeat for several breaths, alternating nostrils with each inhale and exhale.

Breath Control Techniques in Chair Yoga

In addition to breath awareness techniques, there are several techniques that can be used to control the breath in chair yoga practice. Here are a few techniques to try:

1. Counted Breathing

Counted breathing is a technique that involves counting the length of your inhales and exhales to create a consistent rhythm and pace. To practice counted breathing, sit comfortably in your chair with your feet flat on the ground and your hands resting on your thighs. Inhale deeply for a count of four, then hold the breath for a count of four. Exhale slowly for a count of four, then hold the breath for a count of four. Repeat for several breaths, focusing on the rhythm and pace of the breath.

2. Breath Retention

Breath retention is a technique that involves holding the breath for a brief period of time after inhaling or exhaling. This technique can help to increase lung capacity and improve respiratory function. To practice breath retention, sit comfortably in your chair with your feet flat on the ground and your hands resting on your thighs. Inhale deeply, then hold the breath for a count of four. Exhale slowly, then hold the breath out for a count of four. Repeat for several breaths, gradually increasing the length of the breath retention as you become more comfortable with the technique.

3. Kapalabhati Breathing

Kapalabhati breathing is a technique that involves short, forceful exhales followed by passive inhales. This technique can help to energize the body and improve circulation. To practice kapalabhati breathing, sit comfortably in your chair with your feet flat on the ground and your hands resting on your thighs. Inhale deeply, then exhale forcefully through your nose while pulling your belly in towards your spine. Allow the inhale to happen passively, without effort. Repeat for several breaths, gradually increasing the pace and intensity of the exhales.

Incorporating Breath Work into Chair Yoga Practice

Breath work can be incorporated into chair yoga practice in several ways. Here are a few techniques to try:

1. Breath Awareness During Asanas

As you move through chair yoga asanas, focus on maintaining steady, even breath. Breathe deeply into the belly as you inhale, and exhale slowly and steadily. This can help to improve posture and spinal alignment and increase your awareness of your breath and your body.

2. Pranayama Practice

Dedicate a portion of your chair yoga practice to pranayama, or breath work. Choose one or more of the techniques outlined above and practice for several minutes, focusing on the sensations of the breath and the effects of the practice on your body and mind.

3. Guided Meditation

Incorporate guided meditation into your chair yoga practice, focusing on breath awareness and control. Use a guided meditation that emphasizes deep breathing and relaxation and allow yourself to sink into a state of calm and peacefulness.

Breath awareness and control are integral components of chair yoga practice for seniors. By incorporating breath work into your practice, you can improve your mental and physical wellbeing, increase your awareness of your body and breath, and deepen your yoga practice. Experiment with different breath awareness and control techniques and find the ones that work best for you and your body.

Chapter 8: Seated Warm-Up Exercises

Seated warm-up exercises are an essential part of any chair yoga practice. They help to prepare the body for movement, increase circulation, and loosen up tight muscles and joints. In this chapter, we will explore some simple and effective seated warm-up exercises that are ideal for seniors.

1. Neck Rolls

Neck rolls are a great way to warm up the neck and shoulders, and release tension in these areas. To practice neck rolls, sit comfortably in your chair with your feet flat on the ground and your hands resting on your thighs. Slowly lower your chin to your chest, and roll your head to the right, bringing your ear towards your right shoulder. Hold for a few breaths, then roll your head back to centre, and repeat on the left side. Continue rolling your head from side to side for several repetitions, breathing deeply and smoothly.

2. Shoulder Shrugs

Shoulder shrugs are a simple and effective way to warm up the shoulders and upper back. To practice shoulder shrugs, sit comfortably in your chair with your feet flat on the ground and your hands resting on your thighs. Inhale deeply, then shrug your shoulders up towards your ears. Hold for a few breaths, then exhale and release the shoulders down. Repeat for several repetitions, focusing on releasing tension in the shoulders and upper back.

3. Wrist Circles

Wrist circles are a gentle way to warm up the wrists and hands and improve circulation in these areas. To practice wrist circles, sit comfortably in your chair with your feet flat on the ground and your hands resting on your thighs. Extend your right arm out in front of you, and rotate your wrist in a circular motion, moving the hand in a clockwise direction. Repeat for several repetitions, then switch to the left wrist and rotate in a counter clockwise direction.

4. Ankle Circles

Ankle circles are a great way to warm up the ankles and feet and improve circulation in these areas. To practice ankle circles, sit comfortably in your chair with your feet flat on the ground. Lift your right foot off the ground, and rotate your ankle in a circular motion, moving the foot in a clockwise direction. Repeat for several repetitions, then switch to the left ankle and rotate in a counter clockwise direction.

5. Spinal Twist

Spinal twists are an excellent way to warm up the spine and improve mobility in the back. To practice a seated spinal twist, sit comfortably in your chair with your feet flat on the ground and your hands resting on your thighs. Inhale deeply, then exhale and twist to the right, placing your left hand on the outside of your right thigh and your right hand on the back of the chair. Hold for a few breaths, then inhale and release the twist. Repeat on the left side, twisting to the left and placing your right hand on the outside of your left thigh and your left hand on the back of the chair.

Incorporating Seated Warm-Up Exercises into Chair Yoga Practice

Seated warm-up exercises can be incorporated into chair yoga practice in several ways. Here are a few tips to keep in mind:

1. Begin Your Practice with Warm-Ups

Start your chair yoga practice with a few minutes of seated warm-up exercises to prepare your body for movement.

2. Focus on Gentle Movements

Remember to keep your movements gentle and smooth, avoiding any sudden or jerky motions that could cause injury.

3. Listen to Your Body

Pay attention to your body's sensations as you practice and modify or skip any movements that don't feel comfortable or safe for you.

4. Use Props as Needed

Don't hesitate to use props like blankets, blocks, or straps to support your body and make the warm-up exercises more accessible.

5. Breathe Mindfully

As you practice the seated warm-up exercises, remember to focus on your breath. Inhale deeply through your nose, and exhale smoothly through your mouth. Try to synchronize your movements with your breath and use your breath to release tension and promote relaxation.

6. Repeat Movements as Needed

If you find a particular warm-up exercise helpful, feel free to repeat it several times. Repetition can help to deepen your body's awareness of the movement and increase its benefits.

7. End with a Relaxation Pose

After completing your warm-up exercises, take a few moments to rest in a relaxation pose like Savasana. This will allow your body and mind to fully relax and prepare for the rest of your chair yoga practice.

By incorporating these simple seated warm-up exercises into your chair yoga practice, you can improve your flexibility, mobility, and overall wellbeing. These exercises are gentle, effective, and accessible for seniors of all levels of fitness and experience. So, take a few moments to warm up your body before your next chair yoga practice, and feel the difference in your mind and body!

Chapter 9: Seated Sun Salutations

Sun Salutations, also known as Surya Namaskar, are a series of flowing yoga postures traditionally performed as a way to greet and honor the sun. The Sun Salutation sequence is typically performed standing, but it can also be adapted for seated chair yoga practice. In this chapter, we will explore the benefits and steps of Seated Sun Salutations, a modified version of the traditional sequence suitable for seniors and those with limited mobility.

Benefits of Seated Sun Salutations

Seated Sun Salutations offer numerous benefits for seniors, including:

1. Increased Flexibility: Seated Sun Salutations involve stretching and moving the body through various positions, which helps to increase flexibility and range of motion.

2. Improved Circulation: The flowing movements of Seated Sun Salutations can help to increase blood flow and circulation throughout the body.

3. Boosted Energy: Sun Salutations are traditionally performed in the morning to awaken the body and mind. Seniors can also benefit from the energizing effects of Seated Sun Salutations, which can help to improve mood and mental clarity.

4. Strengthened Muscles: The various postures of Seated Sun Salutations engage different muscle groups, helping to tone and strengthen the body.

5.

Steps of Seated Sun Salutations

Here is a step-by-step guide to Seated Sun Salutations:

1. Begin in Mountain Pose: Sit up tall in your chair with your feet flat on the ground and your hands resting on your thighs.

2. Inhale and Raise Your Arms: As you inhale, lift your arms up overhead, stretching your fingertips towards the sky.

3. Exhale and Forward Fold: As you exhale, fold forward from your hips, reaching your hands towards your feet or the ground. Allow your head and neck to relax.

4. Inhale and Look Up: On your next inhale, lift your chest and head up towards the sky, lengthening your spine.

5. Exhale and Round Your Back: As you exhale, round your spine and bring your chin towards your chest.

6. Inhale and Return to Mountain Pose: On your next inhale, sit up tall and lift your arms up overhead, returning to Mountain Pose.

7. Repeat Steps 2-6: Repeat Steps 2-6 for several rounds, moving smoothly and continuously with your breath.

8. End in Mountain Pose: Finish in Mountain Pose, taking a few deep breaths before moving on to your next chair yoga pose or relaxation.

Tips for Practicing Seated Sun Salutations

Here are a few tips to help you get the most out of your Seated Sun Salutations practice:

1. Focus on Your Breath: As with any yoga practice, the breath is key. Try to synchronize your movements with your breath

and use your breath to help you move smoothly and easily through each posture.

2. Move Mindfully: Take your time and move slowly through each posture. Listen to your body and avoid any movements that cause pain or discomfort.

3. Use Props: If you need extra support, use props like blocks or blankets to help modify the postures.

4. Start Slow: If you are new to Seated Sun Salutations or chair yoga in general, start with just a few rounds and gradually work your way up to more.

Seated Sun Salutations are a great way to warm up the body and mind, and to reap the benefits of a traditional yoga sequence in a modified form. With practice, Seated Sun Salutations can help seniors to improve their flexibility, circulation, and overall wellbeing.

Chapter 10: Seated Standing Poses

Standing poses are a staple of traditional yoga practice, but they can be challenging for seniors or those with limited mobility. However, with some modifications, many standing poses can be adapted for chair yoga practice. In this chapter, we will explore Seated Standing Poses, which provide the same benefits as traditional standing poses while being accessible and safe for seniors.

Benefits of Seated Standing Poses

Seated Standing Poses offer numerous benefits for seniors, including:

1. Improved Balance: Standing poses challenge balance and stability and Seated Standing Poses can help to improve balance while reducing the risk of falls.

2. Increased Strength: Seated Standing Poses engage the lower body muscles, helping to strengthen the legs, hips, and core.

3. Improved Posture: Many seniors experience posture issues due to a sedentary lifestyle or conditions like osteoporosis. Seated Standing Poses can help to improve posture by strengthening the muscles that support the spine and promoting alignment.

4. Enhanced Mood: Seated Standing Poses can help to improve mood and reduce stress by promoting relaxation and deep breathing.

Seated Standing Poses

1. Seated Mountain Pose: Begin by sitting up tall in your chair, with your feet flat on the ground and your hands resting on your thighs. Focus on grounding down through your sit bones and lengthening up through your spine. Take several deep breaths in this pose, imagining yourself as a strong and steady mountain.

2. Seated Forward Fold: From Seated Mountain Pose, inhale and raise your arms overhead, then exhale and fold forward from your hips, reaching your hands towards the ground or your feet. Allow your head and neck to relax and take several deep breaths in this pose.

3. Seated Chair Pose: From Seated Forward Fold, inhale and sit up tall, then exhale and bend your knees, bringing your thighs parallel to the ground. Raise your arms overhead and hold this pose for several breaths, feeling the strength in your legs and core.

4. Seated Warrior II Pose: From Seated Chair Pose, inhale and lift your right arm up overhead, then exhale and sweep it down towards your right leg as you turn your torso to the right. Reach your left arm out to the side, parallel to the ground. Hold this pose for several breaths, feeling the stretch in your side body and the strength in your legs.

5. Seated Warrior III Pose: From Seated Warrior II Pose, inhale and lift your left leg up off the ground, extending it straight out behind you. Reach your arms forward, parallel to the ground. Hold this pose for several breaths, feeling the strength in your standing leg and the length in your spine.

6. Seated Tree Pose: From Seated Warrior III Pose, lower your left foot to the ground and bring the sole of your foot to rest on your right inner thigh. Bring your hands to your heart centre and hold this pose for several breaths, feeling the strength and balance in your standing leg.

7. Seated Half-Moon Pose: From Seated Tree Pose, inhale and raise your left arm up overhead, then exhale and bend to the right, reaching your left hand towards the ground or your right leg. Reach your right arm up towards the sky. Hold this pose for several breaths, feeling the stretch in your side body and the strength in your legs.

8. Seated Triangle Pose: From Seated Half-Moon Pose, inhale and straighten your torso, then exhale and reach your left hand down towards the ground or your right leg as you extend your right arm up towards the sky. Hold this pose for several breaths, feeling the stretch in your side body and the strength in your legs.

Tips for Practicing Seated Standing Poses

When practicing Seated Standing Poses, it's important to listen to your body and make modifications as needed. Here are some tips to help you get the most out of your practice:

1. Use a sturdy chair: Choose a chair that is stable and supportive, with a backrest and armrests.

2. Wear comfortable clothing: Wear loose, comfortable clothing that allows you to move freely.

3. Warm up first: Begin with some seated warm-up exercises to prepare your body for the standing poses.

4. Use props if needed: You can use blocks or a strap to modify the poses if needed.

5. Stay within your range of motion: Only go as far into the poses as feels comfortable for your body. Avoid any pain or discomfort.

6. Breathe deeply: Remember to breathe deeply and fully throughout your practice, inhaling and exhaling through your nose.

7. Rest when needed: Take breaks or rest in between poses if needed, and don't push yourself too hard.

Seated Standing Poses provide a safe and accessible way for seniors to enjoy the benefits of traditional standing poses. These poses can help to improve balance, strength, posture, and mood, and can be modified to suit individual needs and abilities. By practicing Seated Standing Poses regularly, seniors can improve their overall health and well-being, while enjoying the many benefits of yoga.

Chapter 11: Seated Twists and Backbends

Seated Twists and Backbends are beneficial poses for seniors as they help to improve spinal flexibility and mobility, which can reduce pain and stiffness in the back, neck, and shoulders. These poses also help to stretch and strengthen the muscles of the core, hips, and legs, improving overall balance and stability.

Seated Twists

Seated Twists involve twisting the spine while seated in a chair. Here's how to practice Seated Twists:

1. Begin by sitting up tall in your chair, with your feet flat on the floor and your hands resting on your knees.

2. Inhale deeply, and on your exhale, twist your torso to the right, using your hands to gently guide you.

3. Hold the twist for a few breaths, taking deep inhales and exhales through your nose.

4. Inhale back to centre, and exhale as you twist to the left, holding the pose for a few breaths.

5. Repeat the twist several times on each side, focusing on lengthening your spine with each inhale and deepening the twist with each exhale.

Modifications: If you have limited mobility or flexibility, you can use a strap or towel to help you twist deeper into the pose. You can also practice Seated Twists with your feet on the floor or crossed at the ankles.

Benefits: Seated Twists can help to improve spinal mobility and flexibility, increase circulation to the internal organs, and stimulate digestion.

Seated Backbends

Seated Backbends involve arching the spine backwards while seated in a chair. Here's how to practice Seated Backbends:

1. Sit up tall in your chair, with your feet flat on the floor and your hands resting on your thighs.

2. Inhale deeply, and on your exhale, arch your spine backwards, lifting your chest and head towards the ceiling.

3. Hold the pose for a few breaths, taking deep inhales and exhales through your nose.

4. Inhale as you come back to centre, and repeat the backbend several times, focusing on opening up the chest and shoulders.

Modifications: If you have limited mobility or flexibility, you can use a pillow or cushion behind your back to support your spine as you arch backwards. You can also practice Seated Backbends with your hands on your hips or the armrests of the chair.

Benefits: Seated Backbends can help to improve spinal flexibility, open up the chest and shoulders, and improve posture.

Precautions: Seniors with osteoporosis or spinal injuries should avoid deep backbends and speak with a healthcare provider before practicing Seated Backbends.

Seated Twists and Backbends are beneficial poses for seniors to incorporate into their yoga practice. These poses can help to improve spinal flexibility and mobility, reduce pain and stiffness, and improve overall balance and stability. By practicing Seated Twists and Backbends regularly, seniors can enjoy the many benefits of these poses, while adapting them to their individual needs and abilities.

Chapter 12: Seated Hip Openers

Seated Hip Openers are an important part of a chair yoga practice for seniors. These poses help to increase flexibility in the hips, reduce tension in the lower back, and improve overall posture and balance. Hip openers can also provide relief from hip pain and stiffness caused by conditions such as arthritis or bursitis.

Here are some Seated Hip Openers to try:

1. Seated Pigeon Pose: Start by sitting in the chair with both feet flat on the floor. Cross your right ankle over your left knee, making a figure four shape with your legs. Keep your back straight and hinge forward from the hips, feeling a stretch in the right hip. Hold for a few breaths before switching sides.

2. Seated Butterfly Pose: Sit in the chair with your feet flat on the floor. Bring the soles of your feet together and let your knees fall out to the sides, forming a diamond shape with your legs. Use your hands to gently press down on your knees, feeling a stretch in the hips and inner thighs. Hold for a few breaths.

3. Seated Cow Face Pose: Sit in the chair with your feet flat on the floor. Cross your right knee over your left knee, stacking them on top of each other. If possible, bring your right foot around to the left hip. Lift your left arm up and reach it behind your back, bending your elbow so that your left hand is between your shoulder blades. Reach your right arm up and over your head, bending the elbow so that your right hand is behind your back. Clasp your hands together if possible. Hold for a few breaths before switching sides.

4. Seated Wide-Legged Forward Fold: Sit in the chair with your feet wide apart. Take a deep breath in, and as you exhale,

hinge forward from the hips, reaching your hands towards the floor. Keep your back straight and lengthen through the spine. Hold for a few breaths.

Modifications: If you have limited mobility or flexibility, you can use a pillow or cushion under your hips for support. You can also use a strap or towel to help you deepen the stretch.

Benefits: Seated Hip Openers can help to increase flexibility in the hips and lower back, reduce tension and pain in the hips, and improve overall posture and balance. These poses can also help to reduce the risk of falls and injuries.

Precautions: Seniors with hip replacements or injuries should speak with a healthcare provider before practicing Seated Hip Openers. It's also important to avoid forcing the hips into a position that causes pain or discomfort.

Seated Hip Openers are an important part of a chair yoga practice for seniors. These poses can help to increase flexibility, reduce tension, and pain in the hips, and improve overall posture and balance. By incorporating Seated Hip Openers into their yoga practice, seniors can enjoy the many benefits of these poses, while adapting them to their individual needs and abilities.

Chapter 13: Seated Forward Folds

Seated Forward Folds are a staple of a chair yoga practice for seniors. These poses help to stretch the hamstrings, calves, and lower back, while also promoting relaxation and reducing stress. Forward folds are also helpful for improving digestion and circulation and can be adapted to suit different levels of mobility and flexibility.

Here are some Seated Forward Folds to try:

1. Seated Forward Fold with a Strap: Sit in the chair with both feet flat on the floor. Place a strap or towel around the bottoms of your feet and hold onto each end with your hands. Take a deep breath in, and as you exhale, hinge forward from the hips, keeping your back straight and lengthening through the spine. Use the strap to help you deepen the stretch. Hold for a few breaths.

2. Seated Forward Fold with a Pillow: Sit in the chair with both feet flat on the floor. Place a pillow or cushion on your lap, and fold forward, resting your torso on the pillow. Relax your head and neck and let your arms dangle towards the floor. Hold for a few breaths.

3. Seated Wide-Legged Forward Fold: Sit in the chair with your feet wide apart. Take a deep breath in, and as you exhale, hinge forward from the hips, reaching your hands towards the floor. Keep your back straight and lengthen through the spine. Hold for a few breaths.

4. Seated Forward Fold with Knee Hug: Sit in the chair with both feet flat on the floor. Hug your right knee into your chest and hold onto it with both hands. Take a deep breath in, and as you exhale, hinge forward from the hips, reaching towards your left foot with your hands. Hold for a few breaths before switching sides.

Modifications: If you have limited mobility or flexibility, you can use a pillow or cushion under your hips for support. You can also use a strap or towel to help you deepen the stretch. For those with knee pain or injury, it may be helpful to keep the knees bent during forward folds.

Benefits: Seated Forward Folds can help to stretch the hamstrings, calves, and lower back, while also promoting relaxation and reducing stress. These poses can also help to improve digestion and circulation and can be adapted to suit different levels of mobility and flexibility.

Precautions: Seniors with back pain or injury should speak with a healthcare provider before practicing Seated Forward Folds. It's also important to avoid forcing the body into a position that causes pain or discomfort.

Seated Forward Folds are an important part of a chair yoga practice for seniors. These poses can help to stretch the hamstrings, calves, and lower back, while also promoting relaxation and reducing stress. By incorporating Seated Forward Folds into their yoga practice, seniors can enjoy the many benefits of these poses, while adapting them to their individual needs and abilities.

Chapter 14: Seated Balancing Poses

Seated balancing poses are a great way for seniors to improve their balance and stability, which can help prevent falls and maintain independence. These poses are also beneficial for strengthening the core and lower body and can be modified to accommodate different levels of mobility and flexibility.

Here are some seated balancing poses to try:

1. Seated Mountain Pose: Sit tall in the chair with your feet planted firmly on the ground. Bring your hands to your heart centre and take a deep breath in. On the exhale, press your feet firmly into the ground, engaging your leg muscles and lifting your chest towards the ceiling. Hold for a few breaths before releasing.

2. Seated Twist with Leg Extension: Sit tall in the chair with your feet flat on the ground. Lift your right foot off the ground and extend it forward, keeping your toes pointed towards the ceiling. Place your left hand on your right knee and reach your right hand behind you, placing it on the back of the chair. Take a deep breath in, and as you exhale, twist your torso to the right, gazing over your right shoulder. Hold for a few breaths before releasing and repeating on the other side.

3. Seated Leg Lift: Sit tall in the chair with your feet flat on the ground. Lift your right foot off the ground, keeping your toes pointed towards the ceiling. Hold for a few breaths before lowering your foot and repeating on the other side.

4. Seated Warrior III: Sit tall in the chair with your feet flat on the ground. Lift your right leg and extend it behind you, keeping your toes pointed towards the ground. Reach your

arms forward, keeping them parallel to the ground. Hold for a few breaths before releasing and repeating on the other side.

Modifications: For those with limited mobility or flexibility, the poses can be modified by using a wall or chair for support. The legs can also be bent, or the toes can be kept on the ground to provide more stability.

Benefits: Seated balancing poses help to improve balance and stability, which can help prevent falls and maintain independence in seniors. These poses also strengthen the core and lower body, which can improve posture and reduce back pain.

Precautions: Seniors with balance issues or injuries should practice these poses with caution and use a wall or chair for support if necessary. It's also important to avoid forcing the body into a position that causes pain or discomfort.

Seated balancing poses are a great way for seniors to improve their balance and stability, which can help prevent falls and maintain independence. These poses can be adapted to accommodate different levels of mobility and flexibility, and provide many benefits, such as strengthening the core and lower body, improving posture, and reducing back pain. By incorporating these poses into their yoga practice, seniors can reap the many benefits of improved balance and stability, while reducing their risk of falls and maintaining their independence.

Chapter 15: Seated Restorative Poses

Seated restorative poses are a wonderful way for seniors to relax and release tension in the body. These poses can be especially beneficial for seniors who may experience stiffness or pain in their muscles and joints. By practicing seated restorative poses, seniors can improve their range of motion, reduce stress, and promote overall relaxation and well-being.

Here are some seated restorative poses to try:

1. Seated Forward Fold: Sit tall in the chair with your feet planted firmly on the ground. Take a deep breath in, and as you exhale, hinge forward at the hips and fold forward, allowing your head to drop towards the ground. You can place your hands on your thighs, shins, or ankles, depending on your flexibility. Hold for a few breaths before slowly rolling back up to a seated position.

2. Seated Twist: Sit tall in the chair with your feet planted firmly on the ground. Place your left hand on your right knee and your right hand behind you on the back of the chair. Take a deep breath in, and as you exhale, twist your torso to the right, gazing over your right shoulder. Hold for a few breaths before releasing and repeating on the other side.

3. Seated Cat-Cow: Sit tall in the chair with your feet planted firmly on the ground. Place your hands on your knees and take a deep breath in. As you exhale, round your spine and tuck your chin towards your chest, like a cat. On the inhale, arch your spine and lift your gaze towards the ceiling, like a cow. Repeat for several breaths, moving smoothly and gently.

4. Seated Shoulder Rolls: Sit tall in the chair with your feet planted firmly on the ground. Roll your shoulders forward,

then up towards your ears, then back and down. Repeat several times, then reverse the direction and roll your shoulders back, up, forward, and down.

Modifications: These poses can be modified to accommodate different levels of flexibility and mobility. Props such as blankets, blocks, or straps can be used to support the body and make the poses more comfortable.

Benefits: Seated restorative poses help to release tension and stiffness in the body, improve range of motion, reduce stress, and promote relaxation and well-being. These poses can also help to alleviate symptoms of conditions such as arthritis, back pain, and osteoporosis.

Precautions: Seniors should practice these poses with care, avoiding any movements or positions that cause pain or discomfort. They should also take care not to overstretch and should always listen to their bodies and modify the poses as needed.

Seated restorative poses are a wonderful way for seniors to relax and release tension in the body. These poses can be adapted to accommodate different levels of flexibility and mobility, and provide many benefits, such as improving range of motion, reducing stress, and promoting relaxation and well-being. By incorporating these poses into their yoga practice, seniors can enjoy the many benefits of improved flexibility, reduced stress, and enhanced relaxation, leading to a happier, healthier life.

Chapter 16: Mindfulness and Meditation

Mindfulness and meditation are important components of a yoga practice, especially for seniors. These practices can help to reduce stress, improve mental clarity, and focus, and promote overall well-being. By incorporating mindfulness and meditation into their yoga practice, seniors can experience many benefits, such as improved mental health, reduced anxiety, and greater overall satisfaction with life.

What is Mindfulness?

Mindfulness is the practice of being fully present and engaged in the current moment, without judgment or distraction. Mindfulness can be practiced through meditation, yoga, or simply by focusing on the present moment during everyday activities. The goal of mindfulness is to develop a greater sense of awareness and acceptance of one's thoughts, feelings, and physical sensations, in order to cultivate a more peaceful and centred state of mind.

How to Practice Mindfulness

There are many different ways to practice mindfulness, but the basic steps are as follows:

1. Find a quiet and comfortable place to sit or lie down.

2. Close your eyes and focus your attention on your breath. Take slow, deep breaths, and notice the sensation of the air moving in and out of your body.

3. As you breathe, notice any thoughts, feelings, or physical sensations that arise, but don't judge them or try to change them. Simply observe them, and then let them go.

4. Continue to focus on your breath and the present moment, letting go of any distractions or judgments that may arise.

5. Practice mindfulness for as long as you like but aim for at least 5-10 minutes per session.

What is Meditation?

Meditation is a practice of focusing the mind on a specific object, thought, or sensation, in order to cultivate a more peaceful and centred state of mind. There are many different types of meditation, but the most common is mindfulness meditation, which involves focusing on the breath and observing one's thoughts and feelings without judgment.

How to Practice Meditation

Here are some basic steps for practicing mindfulness meditation:

1. Find a quiet and comfortable place to sit or lie down.

2. Close your eyes and focus your attention on your breath. Take slow, deep breaths, and notice the sensation of the air moving in and out of your body.

3. As you breathe, notice any thoughts, feelings, or physical sensations that arise, but don't judge them or try to change them. Simply observe them, and then let them go.

4. When your mind wanders, gently bring your attention back to your breath.

5. Continue to focus on your breath and the present moment, letting go of any distractions or judgments that may arise.

6. Practice meditation for as long as you like but aim for at least 5-10 minutes per session.

Benefits of Mindfulness and Meditation

The benefits of mindfulness and meditation are numerous, and can include:

1. Reduced stress and anxiety.

2. Improved mental clarity and focus.

3. Greater sense of well-being and happiness.

4. Improved sleep.

5. Lowered blood pressure.

6. Reduced symptoms of depression and anxiety.

7. Increased immune function.

8. Reduced inflammation.

9. Improved memory and cognitive function.

10. Greater overall sense of peace and relaxation.

Mindfulness and meditation are important components of a yoga practice, especially for seniors. These practices can help to reduce stress, improve mental clarity, and focus, and promote overall well-being. By incorporating mindfulness and meditation into their yoga practice, seniors can experience many benefits, such as improved mental health, reduced anxiety, and greater overall satisfaction with life. Seniors can start with short, simple meditation and mindfulness practices, and gradually increase the length and complexity of their practice over time. With practice and patience, seniors can cultivate a greater sense of mindfulness and inner peace, leading to a happier, healthier life.

Chapter 17: Using Yoga Props for Support

Yoga props can be incredibly useful for practitioners of all levels and abilities, including those practicing chair yoga. Props provide support and assistance in achieving proper alignment and form, which can help prevent injury and make the practice more accessible. In this chapter, we'll discuss some of the most common yoga props and how they can be used to support a chair yoga practice.

1. Blocks - Blocks are great for providing additional height and support during seated poses. They can also be used for balancing poses, by placing them on either side of the chair for additional stability. Blocks come in different sizes, so it's important to find the right height for your body and practice.

2. Straps - Straps are useful for increasing flexibility and range of motion. They can be used to help with seated forward folds, hamstring stretches, and shoulder openers. Straps can also be used to help maintain proper alignment in standing poses.

3. Blankets - Blankets can be used for padding and cushioning during seated poses. They can also be used for support during restorative poses, by placing them under the hips or head for additional comfort. Blankets can also be used to cover the body during meditation or savasana.

4. Bolsters - Bolsters are great for restorative poses, providing support and comfort during extended holds. They can also be used to elevate the hips during seated poses, providing additional height and support.

5. Chairs - Of course, the most important prop in chair yoga is the chair itself. A sturdy, armless chair with a straight back and a seat that is not too deep is ideal for chair yoga. Some

poses may require the use of two chairs or additional props for added support.

6. Yoga Wheels - Yoga wheels are a relatively new addition to the yoga prop family and can be useful for seated yoga practice as well. They can be used to support the back during backbends, provide a gentle massage for the spine during seated twists, and add a new dimension to balance poses by placing one or both feet on the wheel.

7. Sandbags - Sandbags can be used to add weight and stability to certain poses. They can be placed on the knees during seated forward folds or on the feet during balance poses. Sandbags can also be placed on the hips or thighs during restorative poses to help release tension and promote relaxation.

8. Eye Pillows - Eye pillows can be used during final relaxation pose (Savasana) to promote relaxation and reduce stress. They can be filled with lavender or other calming scents to enhance the relaxation experience.

9. Yoga Straps with Handles - Yoga straps with handles are similar to traditional yoga straps but have handles on either end for added ease of use. They can be used for seated forward folds, hamstring stretches, and shoulder openers.

When incorporating props into your chair yoga practice, it's important to remember that the goal is to support your body and deepen your practice, not to show off or push yourself beyond your limits. It's always a good idea to consult with a qualified yoga instructor if you're unsure about how to use a prop or if you have any concerns about your practice.

In addition to the physical benefits, props can also help cultivate a sense of mindfulness and present-moment awareness during your practice. By taking the time to set up your props mindfully and use them with intention, you can deepen your connection to the present moment and cultivate a sense of inner peace and calm.

Overall, props can be a valuable addition to your chair yoga practice, helping you to find greater ease, comfort, and stability in your poses. Experiment with different props and see what works best for your body and your practice. With a little experimentation and patience, you'll find that props can be a valuable tool in your chair yoga journey.

Chapter 18: Modifications for Injuries or Chronic Conditions

One of the most significant benefits of chair yoga is its adaptability. Chair yoga poses can be modified to accommodate a wide range of physical abilities and limitations. Whether you're recovering from an injury, managing a chronic condition, or simply dealing with the natural changes that come with aging, there are many modifications and variations that can help you get the most out of your chair yoga practice.

Here are some modifications to consider:

1. Joint pain or arthritis - If you experience joint pain or arthritis, you may find that some yoga poses are uncomfortable or even painful. To modify poses, use props such as blankets or bolsters to support your joints and reduce discomfort. You can also focus on poses that gently stretch and strengthen the muscles around the affected joint, rather than placing direct pressure on it. For example, instead of a traditional seated forward fold, you might try a seated wide-legged forward fold, which places less pressure on the knees.

2. Limited mobility - If you have limited mobility, you can modify poses to accommodate your range of motion. For example, if you find it difficult to raise your arms overhead, you can use a strap or towel to help you extend your reach. If you have difficulty getting up and down from the chair, you can try seated variations of standing poses, such as seated mountain pose or seated warrior pose.

3. Chronic conditions - If you have a chronic condition such as multiple sclerosis, Parkinson's disease, or fibromyalgia, you can modify poses to accommodate your symptoms. For example, if you experience tremors, you can modify poses to

include more support and stability, such as using a wall or chair for balance. If you have difficulty with coordination or fine motor skills, you can modify poses to be simpler and more accessible, such as focusing on breath work or gentle stretches.

4. Injury recovery - If you're recovering from an injury, you can modify poses to support your healing process. For example, if you have a lower back injury, you can modify poses to avoid bending forward or twisting the spine. If you have a knee injury, you can modify poses to avoid weight-bearing on the affected knee. Always listen to your body and consult with your healthcare provider before beginning or modifying any exercise program.

Some modifications you can try in your chair yoga practice include:

1. Using props such as blankets, blocks, and straps to support your body and reduce discomfort.

2. Focusing on breath work and meditation as a way to cultivate mindfulness and reduce stress.

3. Adapting traditional yoga poses to be more accessible and comfortable for your body.

4. Exploring variations of poses that provide similar benefits but are more appropriate for your body's needs.

Remember that the goal of yoga is not to push yourself beyond your limits or achieve a specific pose, but rather to cultivate a deeper sense of awareness and connection with your body. By honouring your body's needs and limitations, you can create a safe and sustainable yoga practice that supports your physical, mental, and emotional well-being.

Chapter 19: Partner Yoga and Assisted Poses

Partner yoga and assisted poses are a great way for seniors to deepen their practice and experience the benefits of yoga. These types of yoga practices involve two people working together to perform poses and can be a fun and rewarding way to connect with others while enhancing strength, flexibility, balance, and relaxation.

Partner yoga can be done with a friend, spouse, or family member, and it often involves poses that require both individuals to work together to create balance and stability. Assisted poses, on the other hand, can be done with a yoga teacher or partner who helps the senior move into poses more deeply or with more ease.

Before attempting partner yoga or assisted poses, it's important to ensure that both partners are comfortable with the practice and are willing to communicate openly about any physical limitations or concerns. Additionally, it's crucial to take things slow and start with simple poses to avoid injury or strain.

Some great partner yoga poses for seniors include:

1. Seated Forward Fold: Sit facing your partner with your legs extended in front of you. Reach forward and clasp hands with your partner, leaning forward and stretching your hamstrings.

2. Seated Twist: Sit back-to-back with your partner, crossing your legs and placing your hands on your partner's knees. Inhale to lengthen your spine, then exhale and twist to one side, using your partner's resistance to deepen the stretch.

3. Tree Pose: Stand facing your partner, with one foot resting against the inner thigh of the opposite leg. Use your partner's hand or shoulder for balance as you lift your arms overhead and breathe deeply.

4. Double Downward Dog: Start in a downward dog pose facing your partner, then step one foot forward and rest it on your partner's lower back. Lift your other foot and place it on your partner's upper back, creating a stable, supported inversion.

Assisted poses can also be an excellent way to enhance a senior's yoga practice. Some great assisted poses for seniors include:

1. Supported Shoulder Stand: Lie on your back with your shoulders and head supported by a folded blanket or bolster. Your partner can assist by holding your legs and gently lifting them toward the ceiling, allowing your hips to lift off the ground.

2. Supported Bridge Pose: Lie on your back with your knees bent and feet on the ground. Your partner can assist by placing their hands under your sacrum and lifting your hips, creating a gentle backbend.

3. Seated Forward Fold with Assistance: Sit on the ground with your legs extended in front of you, and your partner sitting behind you with their legs on either side of your body. Your partner can assist by gently pressing down on your lower back as you fold forward.

Partner yoga and assisted poses can be a fun and rewarding way for seniors to deepen their practice and connect with others. It's important to start slowly and communicate openly with your partner or yoga teacher to avoid injury and ensure a safe and enjoyable experience.

Chapter 20: Yoga Nidra and Relaxation Techniques

One of the essential aspects of practicing yoga is relaxation. In today's fast-paced world, where people are busy and stressed, relaxation techniques can be a game-changer. Relaxation techniques not only help in reducing stress but also have several health benefits. Yoga Nidra is one such relaxation technique that is gaining popularity for its effectiveness in reducing stress and improving overall well-being.

Yoga Nidra is a Sanskrit word that means "yogic sleep." It is a guided meditation practice that helps practitioners achieve a state of deep relaxation while still maintaining consciousness. The practice is done lying down, usually on a yoga mat, with the support of props like blankets, bolsters, and eye masks to create a comfortable and relaxing environment.

During Yoga Nidra, the practitioner is guided through a series of steps that involve awareness of different parts of the body, breath awareness, visualization, and intention setting. The practice involves relaxation at different levels of consciousness, including the physical, mental, and emotional levels. This process of relaxation helps in reducing stress and anxiety, promoting better sleep, and enhancing overall well-being.

Here are some of the benefits of practicing Yoga Nidra:

1. Reduces stress and anxiety: Yoga Nidra helps in reducing stress and anxiety by activating the parasympathetic nervous system, which is responsible for the relaxation response. The practice also helps in reducing the levels of stress hormones like cortisol and adrenaline in the body.

2. Improves sleep: One of the significant benefits of Yoga Nidra is that it promotes better sleep. The practice helps in calming the mind and relaxing the body, which helps in improving the quality of sleep.

3. Enhances overall well-being: Yoga Nidra helps in enhancing overall well-being by promoting relaxation, reducing stress, and improving sleep. The practice also helps in reducing the symptoms of various health conditions like hypertension, depression, and chronic pain.

4. Boosts creativity: Yoga Nidra helps in relaxing the mind and promoting a state of deep relaxation, which can help in boosting creativity and problem-solving skills.

Here are some relaxation techniques that can be practiced along with Yoga Nidra:

1. Progressive muscle relaxation: This technique involves tensing and relaxing different muscle groups in the body to promote relaxation.

2. Breath awareness: Focusing on the breath and observing its natural flow can help in promoting relaxation and reducing stress.

3. Guided imagery: Visualizing peaceful and calming scenes can help in reducing stress and promoting relaxation.

4. Body scan: This technique involves focusing on different parts of the body and releasing any tension or stress in those areas.

It is important to note that Yoga Nidra and other relaxation techniques are not a substitute for medical treatment. It is always advisable to consult a healthcare professional before starting any new relaxation or meditation practice, especially if you have any pre-existing medical conditions.

Yoga Nidra and other relaxation techniques can be beneficial in reducing stress, promoting better sleep, and enhancing overall well-being. Incorporating these practices into your daily routine can help in managing stress and improving your quality of life.

Chapter 21: Yoga for Pain Relief

Yoga has been found to be an effective tool for pain relief, particularly for chronic pain conditions. It works by reducing stress and tension in the body, which can help to alleviate pain. In this chapter, we'll explore how chair yoga can be used to manage pain and provide some specific poses and techniques that may be helpful.

One of the primary ways that yoga can help to relieve pain is by reducing stress and tension in the body. When we experience pain, our bodies naturally respond with tension, which can exacerbate the pain and create a vicious cycle. Yoga can help to break this cycle by promoting relaxation and reducing the physical and emotional stress that can contribute to pain.

Additionally, yoga can help to improve flexibility, range of motion, and strength, all of which can be important for managing pain. By increasing the strength and flexibility of the muscles that support the joints, we can help to reduce the strain on those joints and minimize pain.

When practicing yoga for pain relief, it's important to listen to your body and work within your limits. Always speak to your doctor or physical therapist before starting a new exercise program, particularly if you have a chronic condition or are recovering from an injury.

Here are some specific poses and techniques that may be helpful for managing pain with chair yoga:

1. Gentle Twists

Twists can be a great way to release tension in the spine and help to alleviate back pain. In chair yoga, you can do gentle twists by sitting with your feet planted firmly on the ground and your hands on the sides of the chair. Inhale and lengthen through the spine, and as you exhale, gently twist to the right, placing your left hand on the outside of your right knee and your right hand on the back of the chair. Hold for several breaths, then release and repeat on the other side.

2. Seated Cat-Cow

Cat-Cow is a classic yoga sequence that can help to stretch and strengthen the muscles in the back, neck, and shoulders. To do this pose in a chair, sit with your feet planted firmly on the ground and your hands on your knees. Inhale and arch your back, bringing your shoulders back and your chest forward. Exhale and round your spine, bringing your chin to your chest and hunching your shoulders forward. Repeat for several breaths, moving slowly and mindfully.

3. Seated Forward Fold

Forward folds can be a great way to release tension in the hamstrings and lower back. In chair yoga, you can do a seated forward fold by sitting on the edge of the chair with your feet planted firmly on the ground. Inhale and lengthen through the spine, then exhale and fold forward, reaching your hands towards your feet. Hold for several breaths, then slowly roll back up to a seated position.

4. Legs Up the Chair

Legs Up the Chair is a restorative pose that can help to alleviate swelling and discomfort in the legs and feet. To do this pose, sit on the floor with your feet on the seat of the chair and your knees bent. Lie back and extend your legs up the chair, so that your calves and ankles are resting on the seat of the chair. Rest your arms at your sides and hold for several minutes, breathing deeply and relaxing your body.

5. Guided Relaxation

Guided relaxation can be a powerful tool for managing pain and reducing stress. To do a guided relaxation, sit comfortably in your chair and close your eyes. Take several deep breaths, inhaling through the nose and exhaling through the mouth. Then, visualize a peaceful scene or image, such as a beach or a forest. Imagine yourself in this place, feeling relaxed and at ease. You can also use guided imagery to focus on specific areas

6. Warrior I

Warrior I, or Virabhadrasana I in Sanskrit, is a standing yoga pose that is commonly practiced in many styles of yoga, including Hatha, Vinyasa, and Ashtanga. The pose is named after the fierce warrior Virabhadra from Hindu mythology, who was created by the god Shiva to avenge his wife's death.

To perform Warrior I, begin in a standing position at the top of your mat. Step your left foot back about three to four feet and turn your left foot out to a 45-degree angle. Your right foot should be pointing forward. Bend your right knee so that it is directly over your ankle and press your weight evenly through both feet.

As you inhale, reach your arms up overhead, with your palms facing each other and your biceps next to your ears. Keep your shoulders relaxed and away from your ears, and gaze forward or up toward your hands.

Hold the pose for several breaths, and then release by bringing your arms down to your sides and straightening your right leg. Repeat the pose on the other side by stepping your right foot back and turning your right foot out to a 45-degree angle.

Warrior I is a powerful pose that strengthens the legs, stretches the hip flexors, opens the chest, and improves balance and concentration. It is also believed to stimulate the Manipura chakra, or the solar plexus chakra, which is associated with personal power and self-esteem.

Chapter 22: Yoga for Arthritis and Joint Health

Arthritis is a common condition that affects millions of people worldwide. It is a condition that causes pain, inflammation, and stiffness in the joints, and it can be challenging to manage. Fortunately, yoga is an effective way to help alleviate arthritis symptoms and improve joint health.

Yoga can be particularly beneficial for people with arthritis because it is a low-impact exercise that can help improve flexibility, range of motion, and strength without putting undue stress on the joints. Here are some of the best yoga poses for arthritis and joint health:

1. Easy Pose: Easy pose, or Sukhasana in Sanskrit, is a simple seated posture that can help reduce stress and tension in the body. Sit cross-legged with your hands resting on your knees or in your lap, and focus on taking slow, deep breaths.

2. Cat-Cow Pose: Cat-Cow pose, or Marjaryasana-Bitilasana in Sanskrit, is a gentle movement that helps improve spinal flexibility and relieve tension in the back. Start on your hands and knees, with your wrists directly under your shoulders and your knees directly under your hips. Inhale and arch your back, lifting your tailbone and head toward the ceiling. Exhale and round your spine, tucking your chin toward your chest and pulling your belly button toward your spine.

3. Downward-Facing Dog: Downward-Facing Dog, or Adho Mukha Svanasana in Sanskrit, is a popular pose that helps strengthen the arms, shoulders, and core muscles while stretching the hamstrings and calves. Start on your hands and knees, with your wrists directly under your shoulders and your knees directly under your hips. Curl your toes under and lift your hips up toward the ceiling, pressing your palms and

fingers into the floor. Keep your knees slightly bent if you need to and focus on lengthening through your spine.

4. Warrior II: Warrior II, or Virabhadrasana II in Sanskrit, is a standing pose that helps strengthen the legs, hips, and core muscles while improving balance and concentration. Start in a lunge position with your right foot forward and your left foot back. Turn your left foot out to a 90-degree angle and bend your right knee so that it is directly over your ankle. Stretch your arms out to the sides, with your palms facing down, and gaze over your right hand.

5. Triangle Pose: Triangle pose, or Trikonasana in Sanskrit, is a standing pose that helps stretch the hamstrings and hips while improving balance and stability. Start in a lunge position with your right foot forward and your left foot back. Straighten your right leg and stretch your arms out to the sides, with your palms facing down. Reach your right hand down toward your shin, ankle, or the floor, and stretch your left arm up toward the ceiling.

Yoga can be a powerful tool for managing arthritis symptoms and improving joint health. However, it is essential to work with a qualified yoga teacher who can help you modify the poses to suit your individual needs and abilities. It is also important to listen to your body and avoid any poses or movements that cause pain or discomfort. With regular practice, yoga can help you feel more comfortable, mobile, and at ease in your body.

Chapter 23: Yoga for Osteoporosis and Bone Health

Osteoporosis is a condition that affects the bones, making them weak and fragile, and more prone to fractures. It is a common condition, especially in women over the age of 50. The good news is that practicing yoga can help to strengthen bones and reduce the risk of fractures.

In this chapter, we will explore how yoga can help to improve bone health and provide some specific poses that can be beneficial for people with osteoporosis.

The Benefits of Yoga for Osteoporosis

Yoga can be an effective way to improve bone health in people with osteoporosis. By practicing yoga, you can:

1. Strengthen bones: Certain yoga poses, such as those that involve weight-bearing on the hands, arms, and legs, can help to stimulate the bones and improve their density. When you practice these poses regularly, it can help to strengthen your bones.

2. Improve balance and coordination: Many people with osteoporosis are at a higher risk of falls, which can lead to fractures. By practicing yoga, you can improve your balance and coordination, which can help to reduce the risk of falls.

3. Reduce stress: Stress can have a negative impact on bone health. By practicing yoga, you can reduce stress levels and improve overall well-being.

Yoga Poses for Osteoporosis

When practicing yoga with osteoporosis, it's important to avoid poses that involve forward bending, twisting, or extreme flexion of the spine. These poses can increase the risk of spinal fractures. Instead, focus on poses that involve weight-bearing on the hands, arms, and legs, as well as poses that help to improve balance and coordination.

1. Mountain Pose (Tadasana): This is a great pose to help improve posture and balance. Stand with your feet hip-width apart and engage your leg muscles. Lift your arms overhead and lengthen your spine.

2. Warrior II (Virabhadrasana II): This pose can help to improve balance and coordination, as well as strengthen the legs and hips. Start in Mountain Pose, and step one foot back. Turn your back foot out slightly and bend your front knee. Extend your arms out to the sides, and gaze over your front hand.

3. Chair Pose (Utkatasana): This pose can help to strengthen the legs, hips, and lower back. Stand with your feet hip-width apart and bend your knees as if you are sitting in a chair. Lift your arms overhead, and gaze forward.

4. Downward-Facing Dog (Adho Mukha Svanasana): This pose can help to strengthen the arms and legs, as well as improve balance and coordination. Start on your hands and knees and lift your hips up and back. Press your hands and feet into the ground and lengthen your spine.

5. Tree Pose (Vrksasana): This pose can help to improve balance and coordination, as well as strengthen the legs and hips. Stand with your feet hip-width apart and shift your weight onto one foot. Place the sole of your other foot on your inner thigh and bring your hands to your heart.

Remember to always listen to your body and avoid any poses that cause pain or discomfort. It's also a good idea to consult with a healthcare professional before starting any new exercise program, especially if you have osteoporosis.

Yoga can be a safe and effective way to improve bone health and reduce the risk of fractures in people with osteoporosis. By practicing weight-bearing poses that stimulate the bones, as well as poses that improve balance and coordination, you can help to strengthen your bones and improve overall well-being.

Chapter 24: Yoga for Balance and Fall Prevention

Yoga is a great way to improve balance and reduce the risk of falls, especially for seniors. As we age, our balance can become compromised, which can increase the likelihood of falls and injuries. However, regular yoga practice can help improve balance, coordination, and proprioception (the body's sense of where it is in space).

When practicing yoga for balance and fall prevention, it is important to start with simple poses and gradually increase the difficulty level as you become more comfortable and confident. Here are some recommended yoga poses for improving balance:

1. Tree pose (Vrikshasana) This pose involves standing on one leg with the other foot placed on the inner thigh of the standing leg. It helps improve balance, focus, and concentration.

2. Warrior III (Virabhadrasana III) This pose involves balancing on one leg while extending the other leg back and arms forward. It strengthens the legs and core and improves balance and stability.

3. Half-moon pose (Ardha Chandrasana) This pose involves balancing on one leg while extending the other leg and one arm up towards the ceiling. It improves balance, coordination, and strengthens the legs and core.

4. Eagle pose (Garudasana) This pose involves wrapping one leg around the other while balancing on one foot and wrapping the arms around each other. It helps improve balance, focus, and coordination.

In addition to these poses, practicing sun salutations and other standing sequences can also help improve balance and coordination. It is important to practice these poses regularly, but also to listen to your body and only do what feels comfortable and safe.

Other ways to prevent falls and improve balance through yoga include:

1. Practicing on a stable surface: Use a yoga mat or other stable surface to prevent slipping and ensure a solid foundation for your poses.

2. Focusing on alignment: Proper alignment is key to maintaining balance and stability in yoga. Focus on aligning your feet, hips, and shoulders, and engage your core muscles for support.

3. Using props: Yoga blocks, straps, and chairs can be helpful tools for providing support and stability in balancing poses.

4. Practicing mindfulness: Focus on your breath and stay present in the moment. This can help improve focus, concentration, and reduce anxiety and stress.

5. Modifying poses: If a pose feels too challenging or uncomfortable, modify it to make it more accessible. This could include using props, reducing the range of motion, or practicing a simpler variation of the pose.

By practicing yoga regularly and incorporating balance and stability poses, you can improve your balance, reduce the risk of falls, and feel more confident and grounded in your everyday life.

Chapter 25: Yoga for Depression and Anxiety

Depression and anxiety are two of the most common mental health conditions affecting seniors. While there are various treatments available, including medication and talk therapy, yoga is a non-pharmacological intervention that has been found to be effective in reducing symptoms of both conditions. In this chapter, we will explore how yoga can help alleviate depression and anxiety, and we will discuss specific poses and practices that are beneficial for these conditions.

How Yoga Helps with Depression and Anxiety

Yoga is a mind-body practice that combines physical postures (asanas) with breathing exercises (pranayama) and meditation. Research has shown that yoga can have a positive impact on mental health by reducing stress, improving mood, and increasing overall well-being. Specifically, yoga has been found to:

1. Reduce stress and anxiety: Yoga helps activate the parasympathetic nervous system, which promotes relaxation and reduces the "fight or flight" response. By practicing yoga, individuals can learn to manage stress and anxiety more effectively.

2. Boost mood: Yoga has been found to increase the levels of serotonin, the "feel-good" neurotransmitter, in the brain. This can help improve mood and reduce symptoms of depression.

3. Increase mindfulness: Mindfulness is the practice of being present and non-judgmental in the moment. Yoga promotes mindfulness by requiring individuals to focus on their breath and body during practice. This can help individuals become more aware of their thoughts and emotions, and better able to manage them.

4. Improve self-esteem: Practicing yoga can help individuals feel more confident in their bodies and abilities, which can improve self-esteem and reduce negative self-talk.

Yoga Poses for Depression and Anxiety

The following yoga poses can be helpful in reducing symptoms of depression and anxiety:

1. Child's Pose (Balasana): This gentle forward fold is a great pose for calming the mind and reducing anxiety.

*   Begin on your hands and knees with your wrists under your shoulders and your knees under your hips.

*   Lower your hips back towards your heels and stretch your arms out in front of you.

*   Rest your forehead on the floor and breathe deeply into your back.

2. Downward-Facing Dog (Adho Mukha Svanasana): This pose helps to increase circulation and release tension in the body.

*   Begin on your hands and knees with your wrists under your shoulders and your knees under your hips.

*   Tuck your toes under and lift your hips up towards the ceiling, straightening your arms and legs.

*   Press your hands and feet into the floor and breathe deeply.

3. Warrior II (Virabhadrasana II): This standing pose can help increase strength and confidence while also promoting relaxation.

*   Begin standing with your feet hip-width apart and your arms at your sides.

- Step your left foot back about 3-4 feet, turning it out to a 90-degree angle.

- Bend your right knee so that it is directly over your ankle and extend your arms out to the sides.

- Gaze over your right fingertips and breathe deeply.

4. Legs up the Wall (Viparita Karani): This restorative pose helps to reduce stress and calm the mind.

- Sit with your left hip against a wall and swing your legs up the wall so that your hips are against the wall and your legs are straight up in the air.

- Rest your arms by your sides or on your belly and breathe deeply.

5. Corpse Pose (Savasana): This final relaxation pose is essential for calming the mind and reducing stress and anxiety.

- Lie flat on your back with your arms at your sides and your legs straight out in front of you.

- Allow your body to completely relax and focus on your breath.

Incorporating mindfulness and breathwork into yoga practice can be helpful for managing depression and anxiety. Practicing yoga can help regulate the body's stress response and promote relaxation. Additionally, yoga's focus on present-moment awareness and non-judgmental observation can help individuals with depression and anxiety develop a more positive relationship with their thoughts and emotions. There is also evidence to suggest that certain yoga poses, such as inversions and backbends, can stimulate the release of mood-boosting hormones and neurotransmitters in the brain. It's important to note that while yoga can be a helpful tool for managing depression and anxiety, it is not a substitute for professional medical or mental health treatment.

Chapter 26: Yoga for Improved Sleep

Yoga is a powerful practice that can help promote better sleep-in individuals of all ages. A regular yoga practice can help reduce stress and promote relaxation, which can be beneficial for those who struggle with falling asleep or staying asleep. Additionally, certain yoga poses, and techniques can specifically target issues that may be interfering with sleep, such as anxiety, tension, and physical discomfort.

One of the most effective types of yoga for promoting better sleep is restorative yoga. This type of yoga involves gentle, supported poses that are held for extended periods of time. Restorative yoga can help calm the nervous system, release tension from the body, and promote deep relaxation. Practicing restorative yoga before bed can be especially helpful for individuals who have trouble winding down at the end of the day.

In addition to restorative yoga, there are several other types of yoga that can be beneficial for improving sleep. Yin yoga, for example, is a slow-paced style of yoga that involves holding poses for several minutes at a time. This can be particularly helpful for those who struggle with physical discomfort or stiffness that may be interfering with sleep.

Pranayama, or breathing exercises, can also be a helpful tool for improving sleep. Deep breathing techniques can help calm the mind and body, reduce stress and anxiety, and promote relaxation. One effective breathing exercise for promoting better sleep is called the 4-7-8 breath. To practice this exercise, inhale through the nose for a count of four, hold the breath for a count of seven, and exhale through the mouth for a count of eight. Repeat this cycle several times to help calm the mind and promote relaxation.

Certain yoga poses can also be effective for improving sleep. Inversions, such as legs-up-the-wall pose, can help increase blood flow to the brain and promote relaxation. Forward folds, such as seated forward fold or standing forward fold, can help release tension from the spine and promote a sense of calm.

It's important to note that while yoga can be a helpful tool for improving sleep, it is not a substitute for professional medical treatment. If you are experiencing chronic sleep issues, it is important to speak with your healthcare provider to rule out any underlying medical conditions or to explore other treatment options. Additionally, it's important to prioritize good sleep hygiene habits, such as avoiding caffeine and alcohol, maintaining a consistent sleep schedule, and creating a relaxing bedtime routine.

Chapter 27: Incorporating Yoga into Daily Life

Yoga can be a transformative practice that not only benefits your physical and mental health but can also help to cultivate mindfulness, compassion, and self-awareness. While attending a regular yoga class can be a great way to deepen your practice and connect with a community, incorporating yoga into your daily life can help you to reap the benefits of this ancient practice on a regular basis.

Here are some ways you can incorporate yoga into your daily life:

1. Set a daily intention: Start your day by setting an intention for your yoga practice. This can be as simple as focusing on your breath for a few minutes, repeating a mantra or affirmation, or setting an intention to practice kindness and compassion towards yourself and others.

2. Practice mindfulness: Yoga is not just about the physical postures, but also about cultivating mindfulness and awareness. Practice mindfulness throughout your day by paying attention to your breath, body sensations, and emotions. Take a few deep breaths before starting any task and try to be fully present and engaged in each moment.

3. Practice yoga at home: Develop a home yoga practice by practicing some basic postures and breathing exercises in the morning or before bed. There are many online resources and videos available that can guide you through a home practice.

4. Use yoga to manage stress: When you are feeling stressed or overwhelmed, take a few moments to practice some simple breathing exercises, such as deep belly breathing or alternate nostril breathing. These techniques can help to calm the mind and reduce anxiety.

5. Practice yoga with others: Join a yoga class or find a yoga buddy to practice with. Practicing with others can be a great

way to stay motivated and accountable, and to connect with like-minded individuals.

6. Incorporate yoga into your hobbies: If you enjoy hiking, swimming, or other physical activities, consider incorporating some yoga postures and breathing exercises into these activities. This can help to improve your balance, flexibility, and overall wellbeing.

7. Take yoga breaks throughout the day: If you work at a desk or spend a lot of time sitting, take breaks throughout the day to stretch and move your body. This can help to prevent stiffness and tension and improve your overall energy and focus.

Incorporating yoga into your daily life can help you to experience the benefits of this ancient practice on a regular basis. Whether you practice at home or in a class, yoga can help you to cultivate mindfulness, compassion, and self-awareness, and improve your physical and mental wellbeing.

Chapter 28: Building a Personal Practice

While practicing yoga in a class setting can be beneficial, building a personal practice allows you to tailor your practice to your individual needs and schedule. Here are some tips for building a personal practice:

1. Set aside time: One of the biggest barriers to building a personal practice is finding the time to practice. Start by setting aside just 10-15 minutes a day, and gradually increase the time as you become more comfortable with your practice.

2. Choose a space: Select a quiet and comfortable space for your practice. If possible, create a designated yoga space in your home that is free from distractions.

3. Decide on a routine: Start by choosing a few poses or a sequence that feels good in your body. You can use resources like books or online videos to guide your practice or work with a yoga teacher to develop a routine.

4. Listen to your body: As you practice, pay attention to how your body feels. If a pose doesn't feel good, modify it or skip it altogether. Remember that yoga is about finding balance and ease in the body, not pushing yourself to the point of discomfort or pain.

5. Be consistent: Building a personal practice requires consistency. Try to practice at the same time each day, even if it's just for a few minutes.

6. Keep a journal: Consider keeping a journal to track your progress and reflect on your practice. Write down any insights or observations that arise during your practice, as well as any challenges or successes.

7. Be open to change: As you continue to practice, your needs
    and abilities may change. Be open to adapting your practice
    to meet these changing needs, and don't be afraid to try new
    poses or sequences.

Building a personal practice can be a rewarding way to deepen your
yoga practice and cultivate greater awareness and connection with
your body. By taking the time to listen to your body, be consistent,
and stay open to change, you can develop a practice that supports
your physical, mental, and emotional well-being.

Chapter 29: Yoga Philosophy and Mind-Body Connection

Yoga is more than just a physical practice. It has a rich philosophical and spiritual tradition that emphasizes the connection between the mind and body. Understanding these principles can deepen your yoga practice and help you develop a stronger mind-body connection.

One of the foundational texts of yoga is the Yoga Sutras of Patanjali. This text outlines the eight limbs of yoga, which include ethical principles, physical practices, and meditation techniques. The first limb, yama, includes principles such as non-violence, truthfulness, and non-attachment. These principles can guide your behaviour on and off the yoga mat.

The physical practice of yoga, asana, is the third limb of yoga. Asana is the practice of physical postures that are designed to prepare the body for meditation. Through the practice of asana, we can build strength and flexibility in the body, but also cultivate awareness and mindfulness. As we move through each posture, we can focus on our breath and the sensations in our body, bringing us into the present moment.

In addition to the physical practice of yoga, pranayama is the practice of breath control. By controlling the breath, we can regulate our energy and calm the mind. Pranayama techniques can be used to prepare for meditation or simply to bring a sense of calm to the body and mind.

The final limb of yoga, samadhi, is the goal of yoga. Samadhi is a state of pure consciousness, where the mind is free from distraction and the individual self merges with the universal consciousness. While this state may seem elusive, the practice of yoga can help us move towards it by cultivating a strong mind-body connection and a sense of inner peace.

The mind-body connection is a central principle of yoga philosophy. The body and mind are intimately connected, and our thoughts and emotions can have a profound impact on our physical health. Stress, anxiety, and other negative emotions can manifest as physical symptoms in the body. By cultivating a strong mind-body connection through yoga, we can learn to recognize the signs of stress and tension in the body and take steps to release them.

Yoga philosophy also emphasizes the interconnectedness of all beings. The practice of yoga encourages us to cultivate compassion and empathy for ourselves and others. By recognizing our common humanity, we can build stronger connections with those around us and foster a sense of community and belonging.

Incorporating yoga philosophy into your practice can help you deepen your understanding of the mind-body connection and the interconnectedness of all beings. By cultivating a sense of mindfulness, compassion, and inner peace, you can bring the benefits of yoga off the mat and into your daily life.

Chapter 30: The Future of Chair Yoga for Seniors

As the population of seniors continues to grow, the demand for accessible and inclusive forms of exercise like chair yoga will also continue to rise. The future of chair yoga for seniors looks bright, with more research being conducted to support its benefits and more instructors becoming certified in this specialized field. Here are some of the ways that chair yoga is evolving and expanding to better serve seniors in the future:

1. Incorporating Technology: As seniors become more tech-savvy, there is an opportunity to bring chair yoga classes online or to offer instructional videos that can be accessed at home. This can make chair yoga more accessible for those who may have mobility issues or who live in remote areas.

2. Integrating Other Modalities: In the future, we may see more chair yoga classes that incorporate other modalities like mindfulness, meditation, or tai chi. This can provide a more holistic approach to health and wellness for seniors.

3. Personalization and Individualization: With more research being conducted on the benefits of chair yoga, we may see more personalized and individualized practices tailored to the specific needs of each senior. This can help to address unique health issues and conditions, as well as improve the overall effectiveness of the practice.

4. Community Outreach and Advocacy: As chair yoga gains more recognition and support, there may be increased efforts to bring this practice to seniors in underserved communities. This can include outreach programs to nursing homes, community centres, and other organizations that serve seniors.

5. Collaborations with Healthcare Providers: With the growing recognition of the benefits of yoga for seniors, we may see more collaborations between chair yoga instructors and healthcare providers. This can help to bridge the gap between traditional medical care and alternative forms of therapy and improve the overall health and wellness of seniors.

6. Continued Education and Research: As with any field, the practice of chair yoga for seniors will continue to evolve and improve as more research is conducted and more education and training opportunities become available for instructors. This can lead to a more widespread understanding and appreciation of the benefits of chair yoga, and ultimately help to improve the quality of life for seniors.

Chair yoga for seniors is an increasingly important practice that can provide numerous physical, mental, and emotional benefits for older adults. As the population of seniors continues to grow, the need for accessible and inclusive forms of exercise will also continue to rise. With its numerous benefits, potential for personalization and individualization, and increasing recognition and support, the future of chair yoga for seniors looks bright.

Chapter 31: Conclusion

In conclusion, chair yoga is a powerful tool for seniors to improve their physical, mental, and emotional health. It offers a low-impact form of exercise that can be done safely and comfortably in a seated position, making it accessible to those with mobility or balance issues. Through its focus on breath awareness, mindfulness, and relaxation techniques, chair yoga can help seniors reduce stress, improve sleep, and manage chronic conditions such as arthritis and osteoporosis.

By incorporating yoga into their daily lives, seniors can enhance their overall well-being and quality of life. Whether done alone or with a group, chair yoga offers a way to connect with oneself, others, and the world around us. The future of chair yoga for seniors is bright, as more and more people recognize the benefits of this practice and its potential to transform lives.

I hope this book has provided you with a comprehensive guide to chair yoga for seniors, and that it has inspired you to explore this practice further. Remember, it's never too late to start taking care of your physical, mental, and emotional health. By incorporating chair yoga into your daily routine, you can enjoy a happier, healthier, and more fulfilling life.

www.ingramcontent.com/pod-product-compliance
Lightning Source LLC
Chambersburg PA
CBHW031321250726
48656CB00005B/1911